Safe and Proven Fasting Guide:

Six Steps to Safe Fasting

A-Z Guide for Beginners

Help You to Lose Weight, Belly Fat, Cleanse Body Toxins, and Reduce Oxidative Stress

Christopher J. Davis, M.D.

Anna G Taylor

Table of Contents

Introduction: Six Steps to Safe Fasting

Congratulations on purchasing *Safe and Proven Diabetes* Cure and thank you for doing so.

Before your introduction to the six steps to safely fast, let's define what we mean by fasting. Fasting is voluntarily depriving yourself of food or drink for a preplanned timeframe. Of course, for those of you who cannot fast food or drink because of medical issues, then fasting for you might mean doing without something pleasurable for a set time. For our purposes in this book, we're going to discuss how to safely fast food and liquids.

The first thing to determine before taking this journey is to discover whether it is physically possible for you to fast. Since we are focused on safe fasting, we do not recommend that you simply set aside food, liquids, medications, and any physical issues you might have to jump right into fasting. This is neither smart nor effective, and it could be quite dangerous if done improperly.

There is much preparation to the process, from before the fast begins to the time you decide to break your fast, your focus

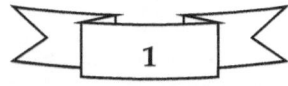

should be first and foremost on your safety and personal purpose for fasting. People fast for a myriad of reasons. They fast to cleanse their bodies of toxins, to clear their minds, to seek spiritual awareness, to heal themselves, to find a resolution, to repent, or to seek guidance and direction. It doesn't matter what your purpose for fasting is; what is important is that you have one.

If your fast is void of purpose, there's a much stronger chance you will not be able to navigate your way through the tough spots and sustain the fast to your planned end. Without a purpose, fasting becomes just an exercise in hunger and sacrifice, and your ability to focus on goals instead of hunger pains will be quite near impossible. Having a purpose or a cause for fasting gives you mental toughness and physical strength. It enables you to get excited about your expected outcome instead of the act of fasting being a dreaded task.

Even for people who frequently fast, it can be a daunting experience. However, for beginners, their first fast can be riddled with pain and pitfalls if they have no supervision, no purpose, and no plan for success. That's why we have provided you with these necessary *Six Steps to Safe Fasting,"* so that you can follow the path of those who have gone before you and end the fast having fulfilled your expectations and rewarded your efforts.

The *Six Steps to Safe Fasting* are as follows.

Step #1: Setting a Plan and Purpose

Step #2: Commit to the Fast

Step #3: Preparing Yourself Mentally for the Fast

Step #4: Preparing Yourself Physically for the Fast

Step #5: Staying Focused During the Fast

Step #6: Breaking the Fast

Many people who begin fasting for one reason end up experiencing results they never expected. For example, you may just want your fast to give your body added energy through a good cleansing fast; however, while doing so don't be surprised if you also eliminate much of that stress and emotional baggage you've been carrying around for some time now. That's the beauty of fasting; it gives you so much more than you thought possible. For many beginners, making it through your first fast is an accomplishment all on its own. Having done what you set out to do should give you a reason to celebrate.

Before you begin fasting, there are some things you should know and expect to happen. The first few days are the most difficult, and they can certainly try your resolve to make a success of your fast. When the hunger pains hit, what seemed like a good idea, in the beginning, becomes something less than wonderful. This too shall pass, but it might take a while. That is why, as a beginner, you must start slowly. Don't go from never having fasted to a 15-day holdout. At best, you are setting yourself up for failure; at worst, you could be setting yourself up for a hospital stay.

Fasting is not a "dabbler's" practice. It requires a heartfelt commitment working toward a worthwhile purpose and making it all happen with a proven plan for success. Food is a basic survival need, and to teach ourselves to do without it for an extended period requires a partnership between our minds and bodies. What our *Six Steps to Safe Fasting* will do is help you align your body and mind with your purpose and plan, so that you can be "all in" with your efforts. Trying to overcome resistance from an unwilling mind or uncooperative body will not allow you to focus on all the wonders you could experience from fasting.

There have been prominent religious leaders who have fasted for world peace, and activists whose fasts brought about a heightened public awareness of ecological urgencies and the destruction caused by global warming. Celebrities have fasted to lose weight for important roles, and physical trainers have fasted for extended periods of time so they could have a healthier, stronger, more energetic body. These can also be causes for you to fast, but in the beginning, your efforts need to be slow and carefully orchestrated for safety purposes.

Another benefit of fasting is that you can do it in the privacy of your own home; you don't have to attend a retreat or make a sizeable investment in products or equipment to be successful. You can fast while you work, making only moderate changes to your daily routines. If you are a highly active person, you might have to modify some of your workouts during your fast. Listen to your body; it will show you your limits. However, the long-term results will be well worth the temporary sacrifices.

Fasting is not something you rush into, so be sure to study these steps before you attempt to put your mind and body to the test, and it will be a test of both. Although we will share testimonials of people who have enjoyed the wonders of fasting, there is no common experience. Some seek spiritual awareness and tell of their communications with God. Others look for a physical healing and report better health than they have felt for years. Olympians who fast have set new world records after having fasted. The more you prepare your mind and body for fasting, the higher your expectations, and purpose, the more likely you are to experience your desired results.

We understand your excitement and enthusiasm to jump into your fast but resist the temptation. First, read through the steps to safe fasting that we have provided so that you can maximize your results.

Chapter 1: Step #1—Setting a Plan and Purpose

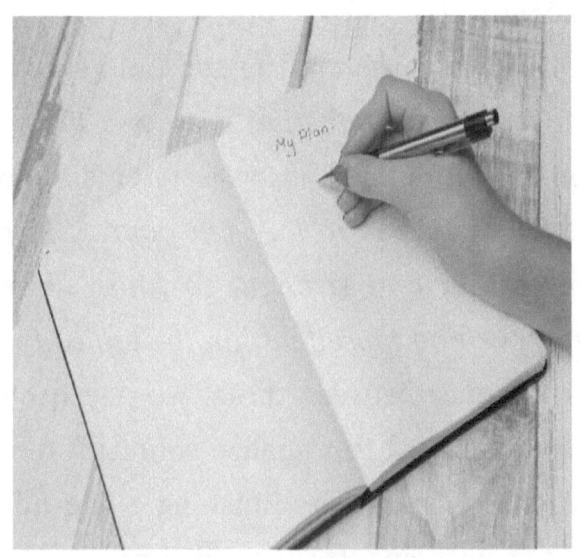

Like almost any other plan, the primary questions you'll need to answer are the "What," "Why," "Where," "Who," "When," and "How," you want to fast. The first step to planning is to decide what purpose you have for fasting. Since this is a personal decision, you will need to give it some thought and then make sure your purpose is strong and meaningful. Since our focus in this book is fasting that is set for a more physical purpose, let's concentrate on helping you state your physical goal in a detailed, specific way.

If your goal or purpose is weak, then your efforts will usually follow suit. So, let's make sure your initial goal is worded strongly and that it creates a vivid vision for your success.

Purpose Statement

A vaguely worded purpose statement would sound something like this. *My purpose for fasting is to lose weight and have more energy.* A well-defined purpose statement looks like this. *My purpose for fasting is to lose ten pounds in five days to gain enough energy and strength to finish June's five-mile marathon and position myself within the top 10 finishers.* Can you see the difference between these two purpose statements? One is so vague it's hard to visualize yourself even completing the fast successfully, much less finishing a five-mile marathon with the top ten participants. The picture is in the details of your purpose statement, so the better you describe your purpose, the more chance you have to achieve it.

Now let's address the six questions to ask yourself to set up as detailed a fasting plan as you have a purpose.

<u>WHAT</u> Are the Perimeters of Your Fasting Plan?

When we talk about the boundaries of your fasting plan, we mean what will be the structure of your fast. To set your fasting perimeters, answer these questions.

1.   What will be the length of time you plan to fast?

This could be quite varied. For beginners, you might decide to fast just one meal at the start. Once you are successful with one meal, move on to fasting two meals, and then perhaps a full day. Don't try to fast a whole week without having had success in fasting for two or three days consecutively.

2.   What type of fast will best suit your needs?

Do you plan on eating no solid foods, and just drinking juices? Or, is your plan to be on a water-only fast? Do you plan on fasting meat, and just eating fruits and vegetables? Some of this will depend on how long you plan for your fast to last. Since you are not fasting for more than a day, for now, it won't matter if you go on a water-only fast. However, the longer your fast lasts, the more difficult it will be to stick to just drinking water. Most people who fast solids, do drink juices and water as well.

Some individuals who are sugar freaks, fast sugar. Or, they give up sugar, fats, and carbohydrates. There are numerous types of fasts from which to choose. It depends on what will best suit your purpose. If you are fasting for strength and energy, then it would be beneficial for you to do some research and see what foods make you feel sluggish and lethargic, and make sure those will be included in the foods you fast.

3.   What impact will your fast have on your family and friends?

This may sound like an insignificant issue, but if you are used to having Sunday dinners with family, then you might decide to begin your fast on a different day. If you feel it is impossible to fast and still prepare yummy meals for your family, then share your plan with them and solicit their support.

<u>WHY</u> Have You Chosen to Fast?

Although the "why" might sound like your purpose for fasting, it isn't the same. To illustrate the differences, let's go back and examine your purpose once again. Okay, your purpose was to lose ten pounds in five days and gain enough energy and strength to finish a marathon within the top ten. Okay, so why fast? Why not just diet or exercise, or do nothing and hope that you'll be successful? Perhaps you've tried all that before and couldn't lose those last, stubborn ten pounds that would make your run so much easier. Or, maybe when you diet, it affects your mood, and you want to run with a positive attitude and a clear mind.

Can you see the difference between purpose and the "why" of your fasting plan? Pondering why you chose to fast gives you clearer purpose to do so. It increases your resolve so that you begin your fast with a knowing that this was the right thing to do to give you your desired results.

<u>WHERE</u> Do You Plan on Fasting?

Because you are just beginning to experience the ups and downs of fasting, you might not wish to fast during work hours at first. Usually, for beginners, fasting at home is your best bet. It allows you to be in the comfort of your home and close to a bathroom. For those of you who haven't detoxed or performed a body cleanse from fasting, you'll probably have a lot of toxins to eliminate. When this is the case, your digestive track can talk back to you a bit, so it's better not to be running back and forth when you're at work.

Sometimes fasting can cause you to be emotional or grumpy, kind of like how you feel when you are hungry and have to wait for your dinner. If your fast lasts longer than a day, these feelings of frustration or impatience can multiply, so it's a good idea to be in a place where you can rest if you need to, listen to some relaxing music, and just focus on visualizing your success.

<u>WHO</u> Will Be Supervising Your Fast?

Will you be under a doctor's care? Will your significant other be monitoring your progress in case you need some assistance? Do you plan on fasting with a workout friend or in a group of people? The reason to ask the "who" of your plan, is that if you should run into unexpected issues, who will you turn to for help? The experiences you are having during your fast might be entirely reasonable, and a person who is seasoned in fasting would be able to quickly put your concerns to rest.

Perhaps the feelings you are having while fasting are depression or disbelief, wouldn't it be a good thing to have included someone in your plan who would offer support and encouragement to help you reach your goal? If you haven't included a "go-to" person in your fasting plan, you won't know who to contact for a much-needed boost in spirit and resolve.

<u>WHEN</u> Do You Plan to Fast?

In the beginning, the "when" part of your plan can be critical to your success. Try your first fast on a day when you don't have anything else planned, and you're out of work. Sometimes planning your fast for just one meal means that you make it your first or last meal of the day. If you are planning a special event or party, that might not be the time to begin a fast, right?

If your relationship with your boyfriend or spouse has been a bit testy lately, you might wish to choose a time when you won't have as much contact with him or her. Remember, fasting can take its toll on your emotions at first, and you don't want to put any additional stress on an already rocky relationship.

<u>HOW</u> Do You Plan to Reward Yourself after a Successful Fast?

I hope you're not saying to yourself that you plan on eating a huge steak and a baked potato as your reward. You've just accomplished a challenging endeavor; you deserve a reward. If your purpose was to run that marathon, perhaps you treat yourself to new workout clothes or running shoes. Even though you will feel victorious for having successfully fasted, whatever you can do to encourage yourself to continue—do it. Maybe you want to get my next book on fasting and advance to the next level.

Another "how" question to ask yourself is—how do you plan on breaking your fast? Just as there is a proper way to begin the fast, there is also a safe way to end it. We'll be discussing this in a later chapter, but just know that you should include it in your plan before starting your fast.

The Importance of Planning

Planning is one of the most important elements of a successful fast, especially for beginners. Proper planning can uncover certain problems that you might not think about until you're right in the middle of your fast and need resolution. Then what do you do? Those unexpected issues can end a fast just like that if you're caught off guard and don't know how to handle the problem. It's much easier to be confident about the decisions you make when you have a plan, even if you need to decide quickly. At least you haven't been blindsided right in the middle of your fast.

Planning gives you all-around better control over your fast.

Your resolve is stronger, your body is prepared, and your emotions are in check. You've consulted your doctor, your fasting buddy, and you have the support of family just in case you're out of sorts for a while. Your fear won't escalate if you should feel a little dizzy or tired because you're prepared for those things. You understand the possibilities.

The Testimony of a Woman's First Water Only Two-Day Fast Experience

Day One—Morning

- I got up at 5:30 a.m. today, which is normal for me. I work from home, and mornings are usually my most productive time.
- Unfortunately, I missed my usual flavored coffee, but my excitement for the fast carried me through.
- I worked until 11:30 a.m., and then began to get a little anxious because I wasn't going to have lunch.
- I continued to focus on my writing, and so the feelings passed.
- I usually have trouble drinking enough water, but by this afternoon I had finished two large bottles.
- Now I'm running to the bathroom every fifteen minutes— pretty annoying.

- It's going on 2:30 p.m., and I'm not feeling any real hunger pains yet. Of course not; it's only been half a day, right? However, on any other day, by now, I would have done some impressive snacking on my break. Oh, and I'd drink a diet soda to wake me up a little.

Day One—Afternoon

- I continue to work and drink yet more water. No problem drinking plenty of water today.
- I usually need to force myself to drink water, but it tastes good about right now.
- Have an urge for something sweet, but I tell myself to get over it. Well, that didn't work.
- I'm starting to feel a slight headache. It's probably due to the lack of caffeine and sugar.
- It's 4:00 p.m.—my favorite time to snack. I'm finding my thoughts preoccupied with food. Wow, I can't even go one day without being consumed by what I consume?
- I wonder how I'll feel when I cook dinner for the family tonight and don't eat anything?

- I haven't been as productive today as I usually am; it's difficult for me to work when I'm thinking about food all the time.
- I'm beginning to feel hungry now, and a little sorry for myself with thoughts of going to bed without dinner.

Day One—Evening

- I ran out of bottled water. Who would have thought I would drink so much?
- I cooked dinner, and it smelled so good.
- My stomach is beginning to churn a little from hunger. A lot of growling going on. It started happened after I cooked.

Day One—Night

- I'm so hungry; I'm just trying to remember why I ever started this whole fast thing.
- Went to bed early because I couldn't stop thinking about food.
- It's 2:00 a.m., and I can't get to sleep.
- I also feel cold, and I'm always hot when everyone else is cold. That's strange.
- It's 4:00 a.m., and I finally give up on the whole sleep idea and just get up.

Day Two—Morning

- It's 5:30 a.m., and I really, really want my coffee—please, could I have a coffee, NOW!
- The water just isn't getting it today, but I know I have to drink it.
- I feel a little shaky, and my headache is more pronounced.
- I'm working this morning, but I don't know how productive I am feeling.
- It's 11:30 a.m., and I think I'm going to take a little nap. I can do that since I work from home.
- It's 2:00 p.m., and I'm just getting up from my nap. Wow, I never take a two-and-a-half-hour nap.
- I had a little diarrhea when I got up from my nap.
- One of my clients just called, and I didn't want to sit and listen to her talk about things I'm not interested in, but I don't know why that should bother me now. She always talks about things that don't interest me.
- I don't think I have near as much patience today, and I'm still feeling tired.

Day Two—Afternoon

- My headache is worse, and I'm feeling a bit nauseous.

- I deride myself for having so much self-pity when it's only been 1 ½ days of fasting.
- Maybe I'm just using my fasting as an excuse for my bad mood.
- I find myself gazing out my window more this afternoon instead of working on my project.
- It's 5:00 p.m., and I am definitely not cooking tonight. The thought of it makes me sick to my stomach.
- I'm still having some diarrhea, and I'm feeling a bit weak and shaky.

Day Two—Evening

- I need to go to the grocery store, but I don't want to make a list of all the food I can't have.
- I went to the store. It sucked! One thing I did notice, though, was that I could smell lots of food in the store. Usually, I just rush on through.
- I took my time shopping and took big, long sniffs of food. I think it was like a teaser "scratch and sniff" test.
- The family brought in pizza. I told them to do what they wanted to do about dinner. What was I thinking?

- It's 8:00 p.m. and nobody cleaned up the leftover pizza off the counter. I want to sneak a piece of it. Even the already been chewed slices look good.
- My stomach is growling so loud I woke the dog. How embarrassing.
- It's 9:30 p.m., and I just want to curl up and go to bed, so I don't have to think about food anymore

Day Two—Night
- I can't wait until morning to have some juice and perhaps a piece of toast.
- It's 1:30 a.m., and I'm so tired. I'm thankful I can sleep tonight, so I don't have to think about my hunger.
- It's 3:30 a.m., and my hunger pains woke me up.
- Morning—where are you?!!!

It's 5:30 a.m.—END OF FAST!!

This was the first-time fasting experience of a 50-year-old woman. Although she is overweight, her doctor told her she was healthy and allowed to participate in the fast. Some of her comments after the fast were as follows.

- Looking back over the little journal I kept during my fast, I was surprised at how much I was focused on food and my hunger instead of all the goals and purpose I had planned.

- The one thing it did for me was that it helped me to drink more water. Oh, and I dropped a few pounds.

- My headaches went away, and I think I'm going to try to stay away from caffeine. I'll probably feel better, and that's a good thing.

- To be quite honest with you, I decided to fast because a friend asked me to do it with her. My purpose was simply to please her and get through it. After reading your book, I do think it would have been much easier for me had a planned a stronger purpose.

- I think I would fast again. It wasn't so bad. One thing I would do, though, is drink juices instead of just water. I think that would give me more energy and focus.

Chapter 2: Step #2—Commit to the Fast

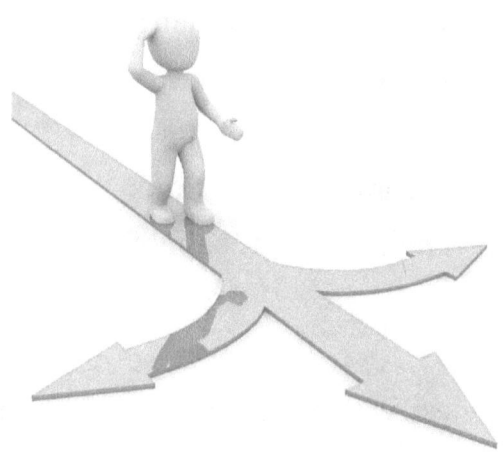

It's so much easier to make a commitment than to keep a commitment, isn't it? You can prepare so well for your fast and your commitment seems so strong, and then right in the middle of it, everything can fall apart. Why? Was the initial commitment not genuine enough or strong enough to sustain the fast? Perhaps! Did you suddenly change your mind when you were distracted by chaotic emotions and a deep physical need for food? Maybe!

Most of all, you are human, and humans often make

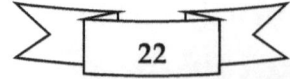

commitments they do not keep. The beauty of being a human with flawed promises is that if we were honest with ourselves and one another, we could all relate to your imperfections. I doubt that you could find one person who has successfully fasted for a long time that could say they never quit a fast. The difference in those who can work through a strict fast is that they have managed to find success in their failures. They have learned from them and taught others because they made themselves vulnerable by sharing their failure lessons. Showing your flaws helps others to relate to you and to understand themselves better.

Reaching a final success is almost always shadowed by failures. For this reason, it's helpful to look at every attempt to fast as a personal stretch to a higher level of success. If you planned to fast for a week and only made it through two days, that's okay. Think of it as a successful two-day fast. Then, make a commitment to plan a three-day fast again later. That's a commitment—to fast after a failed attempt. Think of it as a new opportunity to succeed. The harder the fasting challenge, the more you will learn and teach others.

Changing Your Perspective about Fasting

Ages ago, people looked at fasting as a form of supreme

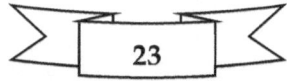

sacrificing, as a punishment even. Fasting was a way to rid their bodies of carnal needs and spiritual temptations. In fact, fasting was often coupled with flogging as a form of self-punishment. It's no wonder many people perceive fasting as a negative, available to those who prefer self-deprivation to self-acceptance and forgiveness. They've never thought of fasting as a way to gain greater insight and knowledge, to bring about physical and emotional healing, or as a way to increase strength and energy.

So, before you make a commitment to fast, pause for a few moments to consider how you feel about fasting. Does the thought of fasting excite you? Do you anticipate positive changes to happen after having successfully fasted? If you cannot see fasting in a positive light, then perhaps it is not for you. Fasting is to some like running a marathon is to others. Some people have not experienced the altered state one moves into when they are a few miles into a long marathon. They have never felt first-hand the new rhythm and satisfaction you get when you let go of the thoughts of how much your muscles are straining and begin to think about ways to live a better life helping others.

Fasting offers that same escape. If you can make yourself stop fantasizing about food and think of a deeper purpose and meaning to your life, the distractions begin to fade away, and your commitment to the fast takes center stage. You get into the zone, and then, without a doubt, you just know you will finish your fast and succeed in achieving your purpose—and then some. It's amazing how your senses become much more intense when you are fasting. If you can't focus on your purpose, concentrate on how you are experiencing the world differently through your heightened sensitivity.

Soon, you will find your perspective changing. Fasting then becomes a privilege instead of a penance. Your fast takes on a whole different dimension, and your purpose grows and expands to include much more than you initially thought. Instead of being consumed with thoughts of your empty stomach, you become empowered by your change of heart.

Avoid Unnecessary Temptations to Break Your Fast

The wonderful smell of food is an assault on your commitment to fast. Since your first few fasts will be shorter, try to avoid cooking if you can. Let your family know your fasting plans, and ask for their support. For just a day or two, encourage them to eat out so that you won't be tempted to break your fast early. As you prepare for your fast, think ahead of things that you can do to help you fight against the temptation to eat.

If you think back to your eating habits, there are usually certain points in the day that you feel like snacking or times where you are hungrier than others. For some people, their hunger peaks first thing in the morning. If they can eat a good breakfast, they're good to go until dinnertime. For other people, they can go with next to nothing to eat during the day, but the minute they walk in from work they hit the refrigerator. Most of the time it's not because we are hungry, but because we are seeking something that food gives us—distraction from the daily grind or a comfortable way to manage stress.

These times will be particularly hard for you during your fast. You have taught your body to expect food during these times, and it's not going to comply with your fast automatically. Think of things you can do during your fast to break these habits. When you fast for a longer time, you are often able to break these habits for good. In fact, some people fast to do just that, to break an old habit and develop a healthier way one.

Watching television can be a terrible temptation when you are trying to fast. When you want to think about other things besides food, it is overwhelming how many commercials you will see that are promoting food. Food that would never appeal to you if you weren't fasting suddenly looks so yummy you want to crawl inside your TV screen and devour it. It's better, if possible, to avoid watching television while you are fasting. This could be a good time to catch up on your reading or practice meditation. Whatever you do, you'll need some sort of escape during the times when you usually turn to food.

Nothing Is Written in Stone

Nothing about your fast has to stay exactly how you planned it. You'll find flexibility to be your new best friend. If you planned to do something to take your mind off eating, and that isn't working—then try something else. Nothing is written in stone. Your plan is not law or a strict religion that cannot be revised and changed to help you make it through something you hadn't anticipated happening. If push comes to shove and you must break your fast, nobody is going to send the fasting police to your house to punish you and report it on the 10:00 o'clock news.

Being flexible in your thoughts encourages you not to judge yourself and others, not to try to label or fix what you are feeling, but rather just to allow yourself to think. When you detach the emotional strings from your thoughts, it's amazing where they will take you. You can question your feelings and change your mind without feeling the pull of guilt or doubt. You no longer feel the need to deny or ignore your emotions because there's no judgment for having them. Soon, you experience total acceptance of yourself and others. What an excellent benefit of fasting.

If you've wanted to lose weight and be healthier, you can focus on doing that through your fast without beating yourself up because you don't look or feel as you think you should. Instead of wondering what others think about you all the time, you have changed to the point where the most important thing to consider is how you feel about yourself. Fasting with flexibility lets you positively examine your purpose, accept how you feel, and then let go of the negatives. It's much like meditation. Many people who frequently fast often combine fasting with meditation to derive maximum mental and physical benefits from their endeavor.

Being flexible in your thoughts opens the doors to positive change. The more rigid you are, the less you can accept yourself and others. It's quite freeing not to feel as though you must judge yourself or fix yourself all the time. You can just enjoy the present and flourish in the now. Your attentions and thoughts can be taken up with more important things than worry and anxiety about what others might be thinking or saying about you. What vanity—to think that others are that concerned about what you are doing or how you are looking, anyway.

When you are committed to fasting, you are open to and okay with change. In fact, change is what you seek. You either want to change your weight, your strength and energy levels, your emotions, your desires, your mental and physical health, and the list just keeps getting bigger. Don't be surprised, though, if what you think you want your fast to do turns into something much deeper and more meaningful than your original plan. That's the thing about change; it's rather independent. We rarely lead change in the direction we want to go. Most likely change steps up, pulls us by the arm, and says "Why not try this?"

Change makes us think about our past and encourages us to consider a different direction for our future. Our choice is to be mindful and pay attention or to ignore the pull of change and continue in the same old day-in/day-out ruts we've been in for years. I, for one, say bring it on change. The more you embrace the possibilities of change, the more likely those changes are to be positive and productive.

There's one thing about being flexible and willing to accept change, and that is you have concluded that you are not the sum total of your thoughts. You are not victim to your thoughts or to change. You are in control. Fasting puts you in the driver's seat of all that you think, do, and say. That might actually be a purpose for someone just trying a fast—to find more control over their choices, decisions, and thoughts. How empowering!

Fasting is Freedom

Once you realize you're not trapped in your fast, there is an incredible freedom of thought that takes place. Giving yourself permission to quit can be the catalyst to continue. Refuse to allow your commitment to fast to become an anchor that doesn't allow your thoughts to float and flourish, with which to expand and experiment. If you are so tied to your commitment that you cannot change, then fasting becomes a drudgery, an empty sacrifice.

Make your fasting a call to free you from what binds you to the things you wish to change. Become a "freedom faster," and enjoy all the advantages to inviting the challenges of change. Then, be encouraged in every step you take on your fasting journey, and let every commitment to fast lead you to the next.

Chapter 3: Step #3—Preparing Yourself Mentally for the Fast

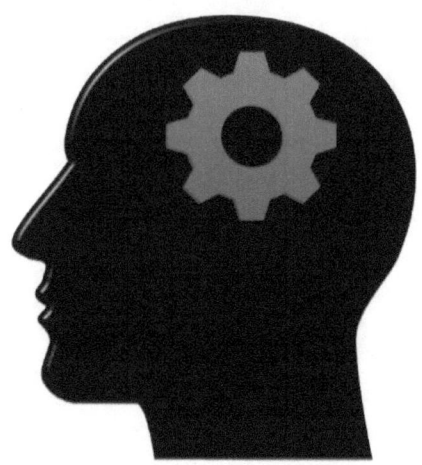

Expect your first longer fast to be an emotional roller-coaster ride. During your smaller fasts, when it only involves a meal or two here and there, you probably won't suffer huge swings in your emotions. However, when your fast increases to more than three or four days, expect the unexpected. The more toxins that are in your body, the more your fast will release them into your blood and the worse you are going to feel. The worse you feel physically, the more your mind will play tricks on you.

For example, on the second or third day of your fast, you might feel so bad that your mind will try to convince you to quit. Your thoughts will be telling you that if something makes you feel this bad, it just can't be good for you, right? Don't give up; that's your toxins talkin'. Longer fasts will strip your body, both mentally and physically, and then build you up to become a stronger, healthier person. The building up is euphoric, but when you're on the uphill climb, you'll feel like throwing in the towel.

The more you know about a longer fast, the greater your chances are of getting over the hump. Once you cross the misery threshold, you'll feel significantly better, but you might not be out of the woods quite yet. Two hours before you end your fast, you could hit another downhill slide that takes you to ground zero. It's all a part of the process, and when you are seasoned at fasting, you grow to expect these ups and downs. Growth is not all daisies and lollipops.

In the beginning, you'll try to keep a tight hold on your thoughts, but doing that will limit your fasting experience. Don't be afraid to give your mind and emotions free reign. Don't try to correct or admonish yourself for where your thoughts lead you. When you give yourself permission to let go, then a hands-off approach is best. At first, it seems like your thoughts have no direction, and that you are just a bundle of anxious energy. However, if you give yourself a little leeway, your thoughts will settle and move you to a heightened awareness or achievement. Like a pendulum that must hit both extremes before finding its center, your thoughts will do the same. They'll go from one extreme to another before helping you find balance.

Why Do People Feel So Emotional When Fasting?

During a typical day when we're not fasting, most of us refuse to manage our emotions. We break up with our boyfriend or girlfriend, and we turn to food. We have a challenge at work, and we head for the vending machines. We get a traffic ticket, and we come home and raid the refrigerator. We eat just as fast and furious as we can until we have sufficiently buried our emotions, whether they were anger, frustration, sadness, confusion, or hurt. We eat, and the emotions subside—then we don't have to deal with them until another emergency arises.

Even though we think we have dealt with our emotional turmoil because it's not uppermost in our minds anymore, we haven't. All we've done is mask the feelings with yummy, gooey, sugary food that turns our attention from the emotions to experiencing pleasure from the foods we are consuming.

Next, we decide to throw a wrench into things and fast. We tell ourselves we're not fasting for the emotional or spiritual renewal, but more for health reasons and to lose weight, right? Okay, but guess what happens? You are made up of incredible emotional and physical intricacies. Our minds and bodies cannot be separated; they're a package deal. Have you ever thought to yourself, "That person would be the perfect partner if I could just separate his emotional shortcomings from his next to perfect body?" The same could be said for an attractive woman. She would be the perfect partner if she were as pretty on the inside as she is on the outside.

Therein lies the dilemma. Our emotions and bodies cannot be divided or separated into neat little compartments, and for one part to be entirely healthy, the others have to be well too. Those of you who are used to burying your emotions are probably suffering from physical ailments because of it. Likewise, those who have abused their bodies, perhaps gaining a good bit of weight, you suffer emotionally because you don't like how you look and feel.

When we have made a habit of burying or ignoring our

emotions and self-medicating with food, suddenly when that food is no longer there to hold down the emotions, everything comes bubbling up to the surface. For that reason, some people cry during a fast, or they get angry and grumpy, or the lucky ones expect the emotional upheaval and deal with all the drama until they get themselves in check. If these emotions have been with you since childhood, and you've suffered under a false belief system, fasting helps you see the truth and rid yourself of these unwanted and unnecessary emotions.

Feeling unstable emotionally during a fast can be quite unsettling when you are unprepared or unsuspecting. Instead of your planned focus of losing weight, you delve much deeper into the cause of that weight gain. If you still try to strictly control your emotions, you'll be cheating yourself out of a healing and a real movement toward good health. So, expect that you're going to have some emotional baggage, plan on how you're going to deal with it, and then let it go and move forward with your fast.

Ways of Dealing with Emotional Stress During the Fast

Strip down and lose yourself in a hot bath or spa for a while. Be as still as you can and just enjoy the warmth flowing over and around every part of your body. Lean your head back, close your eyes, and allow yourself some time to think about these emotions you are feeling. What good are they? Do you need to store them any longer in your body, or is it safe to just kiss them all goodbye? How could these buried emotions be holding you back? How are they affecting your relationships, your work, and your physical well-being?

If you feel like crying—cry! There's no harm in crying; it's a great way to let out the built-up tension and stress. After a good cry, your thoughts are clear and much more positive. If you are angry, think about where the anger is coming from and then let it float away on the water. If it is rage rather than some anger or frustration, it may take more than a warm bath and a round of fasting to free yourself of it. However, at least this is a start, and you are open to the fact that you have unresolved issues that need to be treated so you can live a more fulfilling, happier, and healthier life.

You might feel like taking a leisurely walk in the park to give yourself some thinking time. What you don't want to do is break your fast because you're afraid of the emotions and then keep heaping mouthful after mouthful of comfort food on top of them to keep them under wraps. If you are letting your emotions rule your life, you are not the master of your destiny. You're not in control; instead, you are being whipped and knocked about by emotions that are not serving your best interest.

Once you've learned to fast successfully over longer periods of time, the emotions that surface might be joy and spontaneous laughter. One positive thing to know as you are experiencing these ups and downs is that the deeper the down goes and the longer it lasts, the more euphoric your ups. When your toxins are high, the lower you will feel physically and emotionally. Once you get cleansed, your endorphins will kick in, you'll think clearly, and your energy level will be off the charts.

Imagine the strength of your attachment to food if eating can do such a good job of covering the emotions that are now coming to the surface. No wonder it's so hard to fast for an extended period, not only are you giving up food but you're also letting go of one of the only tools you may have to help you deny your emotions. Now what? Dealing without food and trying to work through these emotions at the same time can be terrifying. I have heard from many a faster who was so overwhelmed with the flood of emotions that he or she refused to experience the temporary pain for the promise of future pleasure.

Contact a Fasting Friend

More than anything, having a friend who has experienced what you are going through helps to encourage you to continue your fast.   When you experience something that frightens or concerns you, you have someone to call.   When you feel as though you want to break your fast, you have someone to encourage you.   When you feel like the fast just isn't creating the results you were looking for, you have someone to give you suggestions on how to make it better.

Your fasting friend doesn't need to be fasting at the same time you are, but he or she needs to be a frequent faster, and preferably someone who is a little further up the road than you. Your friend should know you well enough to get involved with your purpose and know how to help you reach your fasting goals.   It doesn't help to merely have a "yes" friend.   Your fasting friend needs to be someone who isn't afraid to put it to you straight, to tell you like it is. Helping others to heal is more than just telling them what they want to hear.   It's being confident enough to tell them the cold, hard facts about fasting.

It would be wonderful if I could honestly tell you that once you've dealt with these emotions during your first extended fast, they will be gone forever—but, not so. What gets easier, though, is your ability to manage them and release them so that you can heal both emotionally and physically. With each successful fast you experience, the ups and downs will become less erratic, and your confidence will grow proportionately. Who knows, someday you'll be encouraging a faster who is going through the same experiences as you will have during your first extended fast. Take notes, and prepare yourself to experience the transformation from student to teacher.

The most valuable advice? Remember to celebrate each successful fast. Fasting one meal is a success. Fasting one day is a greater success. Fasting one week is an incredible success. Sharing your experiences with a friend and encouraging them to join you on your fasting journey is a success beyond measure. Do you know how many lives you can reach just sharing your fasting experiences with one friend, who then shares her experiences with others, and they help others? It just takes one person like yourself to positively impact hundreds of thousands of individuals. Quite a vision, huh?

Chapter 4: Step #4—Preparing Yourself Physically for Your Fast

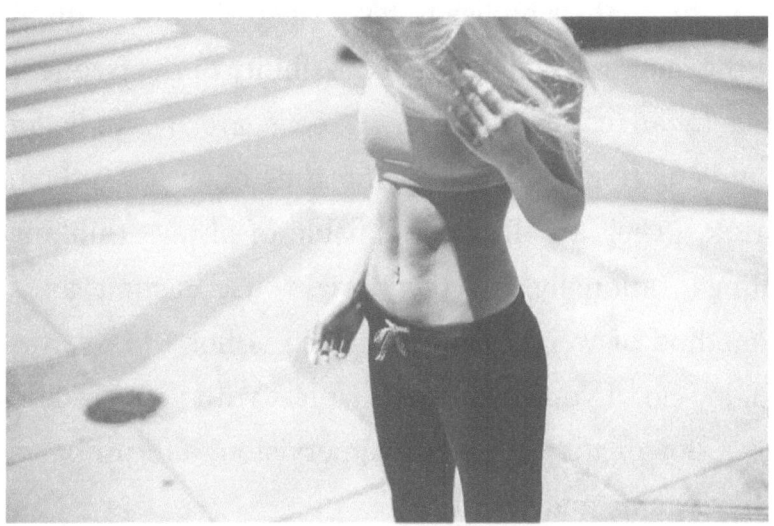

Before we begin discussing ways to prepare your physical body for a fast, let's talk about those that shouldn't be fasting at all. Although this sounds like a matter of common sense, we would be remiss if we didn't mention these important issues. Pregnant women or nursing moms should not fast. Since the fetus or nursing babies get their nutrients from mom, it's important that mom doesn't limit that supply by fasting. While she might be able to do without the calories, babies cannot. Also, children under five years old should not fast for an extended time. The benefits of even skipping just a few meals are questionable, so if you are considering encouraging your children to fast, please consult a doctor.

Teenagers who fast also cause a raised eyebrow. Not that it would be harmful to their bodies to fast, especially intermittent fasting, but the danger lies in the real possibility of the frequent fasts leading to an eating disorder. Teens are a bundle of hormones and emotions. The stress of fasting might push them over the brink. They are also not capable of always thinking through things rationally, so they might use fasting as a continued method of weight control, which is not what it was designed to do. So, if your teen wants to fast with you, I would also consult a doctor for advice and supervision, and probably not recommend an extended fast.

People with heart, kidney, or blood sugar issues should also not fast. Let's look at the fast realistically. You are looking to detox and live healthier, but the stress on your body from a detox can be life-threatening to someone who suffers from these conditions. For them, the roller-coaster ride of fasting is not beneficial.

For those with digestive issues, fasting might prove very useful but also very uncomfortable. If everything you eat moves through you at light-rail speed, and then you create more stress on the digestive track with fasting, the pain and discomfort are going to be significantly increased. For sure, before you decide to fast, consult with your doctor. Keep in mind, if you are fasting because you want to lose weight, there are less painful ways for you to do so without experiencing the ups and downs of fasting. So, you may want to rethink your decision to fast.

Should You Eat a Big Meal Before Fasting?

I've heard some people do this because they think it will get them through those first two to three days of hunger and cravings. Most seasoned fasters disagree. Bulking up on foods that are high in sugar, fats, and carbohydrates are more likely to increase your appetite and cause some digestion issues during the first few days of your fast. It's a much better idea to begin to cut down on your portions and eat less sugar, fat, carbohydrates and fatty meats. Stick to fruits and vegetables, whole grains, and some lean meats as you move into your fast. This will give you fewer toxins as you start your fast, and yet help you feel more satisfied.

Dairy products are particularly tough to digest, so avoid cheese and milk right before fasting. Almond or soy milk could be a substitute, but I haven't done enough research on their effects on fasting. You definitely want to avoid processed foods, especially those with sugar. Experiencing a sugar crash will only make your fasting leave you with stronger headaches—not higher levels of energy.

What About Your Bad Habits?

If you smoke, don't wait until a few days before your fast to try to stop. Fasting is challenging enough, but top that with trying to stop tobacco use and you've got the perfect storm. Quit smoking long before you fast, so you're not going through withdrawals from the smokes as well as the food. Also, if you like to drink a six-pack every night, knock it off long before your fast. Avoid substances like diet drinks and coffee are recommended as well. Addictions come in all forms and believe me; there are just as many people addicted to caffeine as to alcohol, cigarettes, and drugs.

If you are in the habit of staying up all night and dragging yourself out of bed at the last minute in the morning, you may want to rethink this practice as well. Although cleansing your body will eventually give you more energy, during the fast you'll feel tired and drained. Getting plenty of rest is mandatory for a successful fast. It will help you to focus and keep the headaches at bay. In fact, you'll be able to sleep through a lot of your discomfort for the first few days. Allow yourself the privilege of going to bed early and also sleeping in longer than usual.

As for drugs or other substances, there's rarely a good time to do them, but especially not just before you start a fast. If you are smoking medical Marijuana and need it for your condition, just keep in mind that it will increase your appetite.

Water—Water—and, More Water

Depending on whether you have decided to drink juices during your fast, you still must stay hydrated with a lot of water. Not only will it decrease your appetite, but it helps to flush the toxins out of your body. It reduces hunger pains, nausea, and the bad breath that accompanies fasting. Your toxins will be released through the pores in your skin, out through your urine, and your bowels, and you will notice changes in all these areas. Your skin may break out and feel rather oily. Your urine and stool may change color and odor and contain a mucus-like substance. When your body goes into ketosis, you'll notice your tongue will be coated, and your breath will be harsh enough to stop a rhino in its tracks.

The positive physical changes you might experience during your fast are the clearing of your sinuses, a sense of lightness and well-being, and a feeling of renewed confidence and decisiveness. If you find yourself getting dizzy or hungry, try drinking a little more water. Water will be your best friend during you fast.

Drinking Juices

If you decide to include juices while fasting, the best ones to drink are apple, pear, grapefruit, watermelon, and papaya. Preparing them beforehand is a good idea. Squeeze them fresh so that you know there are no sugars added. Vegetable juices are also safe to consume during a fast. Mixing the juice of lettuce, celery, and carrots in equal parts will curb your appetite and keep you from getting listless or lethargic during your fast.

You might also want to include a warm vegetable broth to fill you up and ease your hunger. If you decide to add fruits high in acid, dilute them with water to prevent them from irritating your stomach.

What About Exercising During Your Fast?

Moderate exercise is good, and it helps to release toxins and take your mind off eating, but don't overdo. Walking, and some light Yoga will keep your mind and body busy. Remember, your energy level and focus will be low, especially at first, and your coordination may be impaired as well. Any exercise that is too strenuous could put you in a precarious position should you suffer a bout of dizziness or nausea. A better idea for your first few fasts is to choose days where you have nothing planned, and you can rest when needed, read a book, or do low-impact exercises.

If you decide that walking works for you during a fast, keep in mind that you might need to stay close to a bathroom. When your stomach is empty, everything you drink is going to go right through you, so you'll want to avoid making mad dashes. Those runs to the bathroom might be the fastest you move for the next few days.

One of my friends loves animals and has an annual pass to the zoo. When she is fasting, it relaxes her to go and gaze at the animals, so she chooses a bench near the restroom and sits for hours. Every once in a while she changes locations, always making sure she is near the facilities. It's a way to detox her mind as well as her body, and she always looks forward to sharing her fasts with the animals.

Another fasting friend shared with me how she escaped from thoughts of eating by visiting her local art museum and sitting to admire the artists on display. She gets lost in the art and enjoys her days at the museum. She told me, each time she sits and contemplates the artists' work, she discovers something new and exciting.

These activities have given people who are fasting an outlet to occupy their minds and help them to avoid the emotional ups and downs that can accompany fasts. The outings don't require a lot of energy, but the fasters do get lost in thought and contemplation. They have learned to let their minds swirl and flow in areas that provoke deeper insight and vision than they regularly experience.

Perhaps part of the preparation for fasting is to discover a new hobby that will challenge your mind without stressing your body. Maybe sketching, painting, sewing, gardening, or cleaning your golf clubs or rolling those coins you've been saving. Whatever you do, avoid sports or activities that involve weapons, sharp objects, deep water, isolated areas, or fast cars. Another friend of mine shared with me that she has her daughter hide her wallet because she finds it relaxing and distracting to shop when she fasts. Whatever works for you, give yourself time and several fasts to find your way to success.

Chapter 5: Step #5—Staying Focused During the Fast

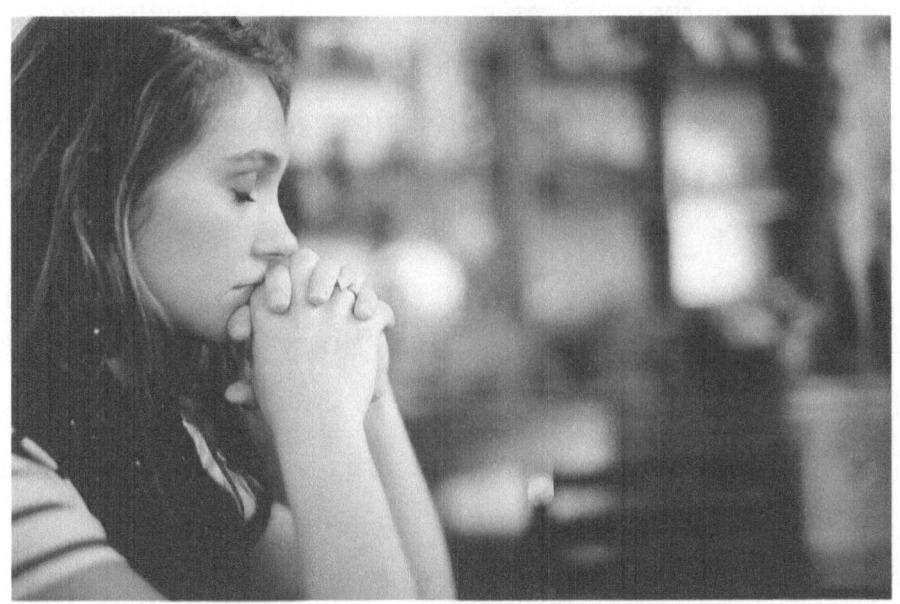

One of the hardest things to do when fasting is to stay focused on your purpose and what you want to achieve from your fast. The danger of losing sight of your goals is that you will break your fast too early and miss out on all the benefits that the fast could have provided. When you're in the first few days of a fast, it's difficult to think about much of anything except hunger and discomfort; however, given time these feelings will pass. Then you must manage the emotional issues that arise so that you can focus on your initial purpose.

Using the tips offered in this chapter will help you focus, but the one most important thing to do to improve your focus and resolve is to make sure you have set a strong purpose. A meaningful purpose will carry you through the tough times of your fast when your mind, friends, family members, body, and everything else under the sun tells you just to quit. If your purpose is weak, your resolve to stick with your fast will be as well.

Five Focus Tips to Keep Your Head in the Game

Once you are confident that your purpose is compelling, then plan on following these focus tips to maintain a positive outlook for a more satisfying fast. The tips are not in any order; you can use them anytime during your fast.

Tip #1—Create a Fast-Friendly Environment

If you're going through all this to detox your body, why not do the same for your mind as well? Don't pollute your thoughts with meaningless television programs. Instead, why not use this time for meditation that gives thought to your purpose for fasting? Before your fast, gather some reading material that relates to your purpose, and decide to seek answers to whatever issues you might have. If you want to improve your work situation, then focus on ways to do that. If you are looking for a meaningful relationship, then use your fasting time to focus on ways you can attract the type of people in your life who will fulfill that need. If you are using your fast to kick start better eating habits, then choose some reading material that will prepare you for that as soon as you rid your body of its toxins.

Without the television to distract you, your thoughts can flow, and your vision will be processed internally instead of postponed by external distractions. The same holds true for background noise, like your favorite radio station blaring the latest wrap tune or even listening to Streisand on the stereo. The noise will block your mind's ability to focus on your purpose and resolve. In fact, anything that involves your senses, like smells from cooking, a room that is too cold or too warm, or loud noises from your children or pets. When you're stretched to find focus, it doesn't take much to dampen your resolve and end your fast.

Tip #2—Get Your Emotions in Check

Even more distracting than the external things are all the emotions playing havoc with your ability to focus. Emotional issues create inner dialogue, or self-talk, that can lead your thoughts down empty and rambling rabbit holes. Most of the time, the self-talk isn't all that positive or encouraging, either. The more negative your self-talk, especially when it pertains to your fast, the more likely you are to break your fast before completion.

The most powerful and influential negative voice in our lives comes from our own self-talk. The experts say that it takes about five positive comments to compensate for every negative one. When our self-talk is so negative, just think of how many positive thoughts you must have to erase the impact of the negatives bombarding your mind during a fast. Not only that, but our negative thoughts stay with us so much longer than the positive ones. We are biased to believing in the negative things we say to ourselves, and those things move from controlling our thoughts to motivating our behaviors. That's why you need to keep your mind active on things that feed you more positives.

Sometimes, to control your thoughts, you must change scenery, act differently, do something that brings you peace and calmness. That's why many people couple fasting with meditation. Meditation allows you to preserve your physical energy while allowing your mind to find sanctuary. Of course, if your television is blaring, or your phone ringing, finding that happy place is almost impossible.

Tip #3—Occupy Yourself with Something You Enjoy

Earlier I told you about my friends—one who visited the zoo when she was fasting and the other who went to the art museum. These were not everyday occurrences for them; they reserved them for times when they needed a special getaway—like fasting. When you are planning your fast, think about a hobby that you enjoy that doesn't require too much physical activity. Set aside time during your fast to do this hobby so that you can distract your mind with something creative, fun, and positive. Make it a hobby or activity that you can get lost in, that your mind can escape all those strong negative thoughts that you are tempted to have during a fast.

I like to take my dogs to the lake and watch them play in the water. I can sit on a rock, get lost in their fun, and soon my mind is peacefully listening to the wind as it blows through the trees and watching the water as it ripples to the shore. It was very soothing, until the dogs come bounding up the shoreline to shake all over me, but even then, they remind me how important it is to enjoy the simple things in life.

Tip #4—Focus on What the Fast Will Do for You

When it's too hard to see all the way to the end of the fast, set up smaller goals so that you will be reminded to check in with your fast and think about what this fast will do for you—both physically and mentally. Instead of thinking about your hunger or cravings, reflect on how your body is getting cleansed and purified, and how you are healing old emotional wounds. Think about how much closer you are today to your final destination with your fast than you were yesterday, or how much better you feel now than you did just a few hours earlier.

If you can't interrupt your negative thoughts or get lost in something you enjoy, this might be the time to take a nap to break the cycle of negative thoughts and bring you back into focus. When you can't get your mind to move forward, you need to change things up by taking action. Go outside and sit in the sun on your back patio, or take a short walk. Another fasting friend of mine told me when she cannot control her thoughts; she finds it comforting to organize something—anything. She cleans a junk drawer in her kitchen or organizes her wrapping paper and ribbons. She goes through the clothes she hasn't worn in forever and makes a trip to Goodwill. Once she feels like she is in control of some external things, she moves back to her inner thoughts.

Consider what the fast will do for you, and focus on those things. What are your expectations? What is your purpose? When you achieve your goal, how will your life be better? Continue to create a vision of accomplishment and then picture that image in your mind.

Tip #5—Find a Creative Outlet

One of the ways to refocus is to find a creative outlet that will not only allow you to experience more positive thoughts but will also help you focus. A great creative outlet when you are fasting is photography. Find a camera, or use the one on your phone, and keep a photo journal of your fast. Along with the photo-journal, write down your feelings. Writing is an excellent way to focus your thoughts. Just think of what an excellent teaching tool you would have if you had a journal of your fasting experiences along with graphic photos.

Another creative outlet is gardening. There's something about growing things that does your soul good. Watching your flowers or vegetables bloom and sprout gives your satisfaction and a wonderful sense of accomplishment.

No matter what you decide to do to help you focus, stay active, and stick to your fast, know that it will take some planning.

Don't wait until you're feeling down and out, and then desperately hunt for an outlet. Experiment ahead of time to see what will give you the best escape and emotional rewards. One gentleman I talked to who fasts regularly has a collection of watches. He never has time to clean his watches, except when he fasts. That's when he'll get out his repair tools and spend the time carefully taking apart the watch and cleaning its intricate parts. It keeps him focused and lost in the activity. There's no time to think about hunger when you focused on time itself, right?

Visualize Your Success

When you can visualize a successful fast and what it can do for your life, it is so much easier to follow through with your plan. Visualization is a powerful tool, and your brain's response to visualization is exactly as it would be if the event you create in your mind really happened. For example, if you cannot get a negative comment someone said out of your head, visualize them in the same place about to speak, but change the message. Change their words by imagining they said something else. It's amazing how replacing their negative words with your positive ones can change the emotion as well.

If you are having trouble focusing on your purpose and all the positive things your fast can do for you, draw pictures of these things. If your purpose is to be stronger and have more energy, then draw a picture of a runner and then focus on your picture. Draw them coming in first in a marathon, and then concentrate on that result. The act of drawing will enable your mind to follow.

You can also visualize yourself succeeding at a much harder task. Close your eyes and imagine you have fasted for weeks. You've passed the rough spot you are going through right now, and you know you can see this longer fast through to the end. You feel light, encouraged, and look back at your current task with the knowledge that this one is easy compared to the one you have already accomplished.

Imagine and create a picture of paradise, where there are no rules, and anything goes. Your imagined paradise has an ocean that is completely clear so that you can see all its creatures. Perhaps your paradise is a place where animals talk to you, and you are filled with amazement at all that you have created there—the colors are vivid, and the climate is warm and welcoming. You feel yourself relaxing under the warmth of the sun's rays, and you hear the waving branches of the palms. See what I mean? Make your visualization as detailed as it takes for you to get lost in it.

You don't have to wait until you fast to do the things that bring positives into your life. In fact, when you're accomplished at dumping much of life's negatives, these things won't be stored as toxins in your body and mind. Then you can use your fast to expand your horizons, to think clearly and creatively, and to create greater opportunities for happiness.

Chapter 6: Step #6—Breaking the Fast

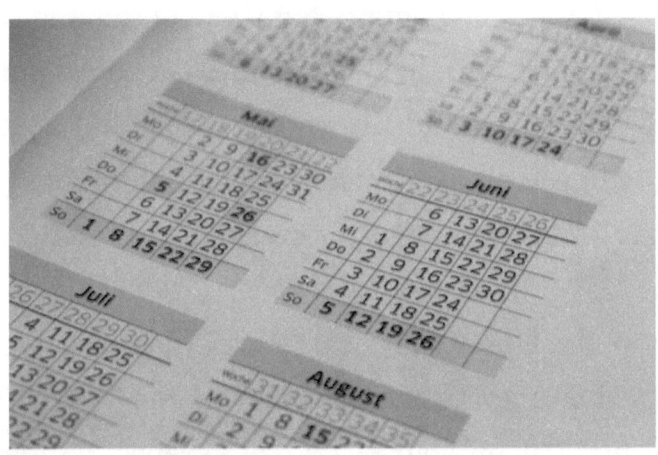

It's so tempting to come off a fast and want to eat everything in the refrigerator, cupboards, borrow from the neighbors, and then make an emergency trip to the grocery store for more. However, just as important as it is to plan for a successful fast, part of that planning should be how to break your fast without suffering severe digestive problems. The key to creating comfort as you break your fast is to introduce solids back into your diet slowly and deliberately.

Breaking Your Fast

Day One

If you have been on a water-only fast, then the first things you'll

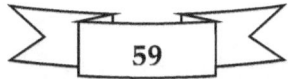

want to start with is some fruits and fruit juices. They will give you some much-needed energy. Avoid the acidic fruits at first until your stomach gets a chance to respond to the other juices. You can also try a boiled potato, but avoid butter and seasoning for the day. Under normal circumstances, a boiled potato with no toppings doesn't sound like very gourmet, but after days of fasting it will be good just to chew something solid. Stick with these things for the first day after breaking your fast.

Continue to limit your physical exercise as well; you're not going to feel like cycling or getting on the treadmill today. Make that first day off your fast a day to reflect on the benefits of your accomplishments and how much you are enjoying the taste of some real food again. Also, don't forget to stay hydrated. Even though you are drinking juices, water will help your sensitive tummy.

Day Two

You can still eat fruits and drink juices, but today add some steamed vegetables to your diet. You can also have another potato, but don't add heavy toppings. A little warm soup is also good, and perhaps a little lean meat like skinless chicken. If these things are too harsh on your stomach, then back off the meat until tomorrow. You might try eating some salad with just a little dressing.

Day Three

Gradually begin to eat larger portions, and introduce more protein and whole grains. Eat less food more often so that you don't overload your digestive track too soon. It should be easier for you to focus on other things besides your hunger now, so take some time to think about how you're going to maximize the results of your fast. Moving forward, begin to introduce more things back into your meals. The last things to include would be anything with caffeine or sugar. Now that you've removed the toxins from your body, you won't want to pollute your body further any time soon.

The longer you have fasted, the more slowly you should return to eating a variety of solid foods. With a fast that lasted just a few days, three days taken to go back to solids will be plenty of time. For those who fast for 20 to 30 days, it could take an entire week to return to normal portions and a wider range of foods. Just getting rid of the halitosis will be a relief.

Isn't it amazing how much sweeter fruits and juices are, and how much more intensely you taste vegetables and robust foods? If for nothing else, fasting enables you to appreciate the flavors, textures, colors and smells of foods you haven't been able to enjoy for a while. Take it all in; allow yourself that time to appreciate and be thankful that you have so many types of foods that are easily attainable. Instead of rushing through a meal, or eating breakfast on the go, take the time to enjoy your food. Be deliberate and selective about your meals.

For a while, try not to add a lot of butter, sugar, or spices to your foods. Eat them raw or natural and enjoy their distinctive flavors. As you add foods back into your diet each day, pay attention to the ones that cause you some digestive issues. Each person is different, so what might bother one will be perfectly fine for another. Whatever foods cause your bowels or stomach to be irritated might be ones that you should avoid altogether.

Did you know that you could have an intolerance to certain foods and never know it? Those intolerances could be the reason you get frequent headaches and have bowel or stomach issues. Many people who are intolerant to certain foods will attribute their body's reaction to the food to suspicions that there was something wrong with what they ate. We're not speaking about food allergies; you would probably have many different reactions to allergies because your immune system would be compromised. Your body would react by breaking out in hives, restricted breathing, and could even go into anaphylactic shock. However, intolerances are much milder symptoms, a feeling that you're getting a slight tummy ache from eating something that disagreed with you.

When you break a fast, your body's signals for foods you might be intolerant of are going to be much more pronounced, so learn to listen to your body. When you are bringing solids back into your daily diet, pay attention to those foods that are upsetting to your system. You might decide to avoid eating them in future or at least limit their intake. It would be an especially good idea to do so just before your next fast.

It is common to experience loose bowels or diarrhea after eating your first meal as you break your fast. It usually doesn't persist unless your digestive track has been irritated by a particular food, drink, or medication. If it continues, it's best to consult your physician to seek relief because sensitive digestive tracks can be painful and sometimes downright embarrassing. Also, raw acidy fruits and vegetables as well as whole grain breads can be high in fiber and tend to add to the problem. Some people consume some probiotics when breaking their fasts, and they've found it to eliminate the irritation and help to balance their gastric system.

You may also feel a sense of euphoria when finishing your fast, which encourages some to overdo the first few days they add solids to their diet. They clean the house, wash the car, mow the lawn, play tennis, and go on an extended hike. When ending your fast, do everything slowly and in moderation. Don't try to conquer cross fit today when yesterday you were having trouble getting off the couch.

When you begin to eat again, make a commitment to eat healthier, less if necessary, smaller portions, perhaps more frequent meals, and be sure to keep it a positive experience shared with family members and friends. Since there is no proof that fasting creates long-term weight loss, why not decide to fast for the right reasons—to cleanse your body of toxins and for guidance and awareness? It's hard enough when you fast for the right reasons, but throw in a little mistaken reasoning and confused expectations, and you have a recipe for emotional and physical disaster.

Fast because you want to give your body a reboot. Fast because you want to gain wisdom and insight. Fast because you want to break old habits and then get a fresh start on better ones. Even fast because you're curious if all the hype about fasting is true. When you do decide to fast, do it safely and slowly, and with forethought and purpose. Do your homework before fasting to find out if it's right for you, and consult a doctor so that you don't do more harm than good.

Don't expect miracles; unless of course, a higher source has directed you to fast and seek truth. For most of us, fasting is a natural thing. Since the days of hunting and gathering when food was scarce, our bodies were designed to function with limited food resources. To stuff our systems with preservatives and toxins is the unnatural result of our century. Less than 100 years ago, there was little need for cleansing and detoxing our bodies and minds. We were used to living in the present and sustaining ourselves with fresh foods that were grown free of pesticides and growth hormones and marketed without the addition of artificial flavors, sugars, and coloring.

Years past, fasting was done for spiritual reasons, somewhat reserved for the faithful and devout. Although most of our focus in this book has been on the physical aspects of fasting, we will conclude with some surprising emotional and spiritual elements to a successful fast. Even if your purpose does not include those things, there's a good chance you will experience a greater awareness of your spiritual side. If you don't on your first fast, look for this to occur on other fasts to follow.

Conclusion: Analyzing Your Results

Testimonials

Grace, 32-Year-Old Woman on Her First Fast

One of the surprising things I discovered after fasting for strictly physical reasons was that I couldn't. Oh, I could fast, but it didn't work out to be strictly for a physical cleansing. I hadn't planned on it, but the emotional and spiritual benefits of the fast far outweighed the physical things I wanted to experience on my first fast. I'm looking forward to my next fast, and this time my planning will include some answers I'd like to receive to issues that have been bothering me for a long time.

Jason, 57-Year-Old Man Who Is Seasoned Faster

I've been fasting for so many years that it's hard for me to remember my first experience with fasting. I was a young athlete in college; I do remember that. I was told that fasting would give me more strength and endurance, and I believe it did that. What I didn't expect that first time, but what I have ever since, is that it is much easier for me to focus after a fast. I have used fasting to visualize wins as I played college ball, and I still focus on winning what I want as an adult. I wish I could say it was easier for me to fast since I've done it so often, but I still feel discouraged at times when I just want it to be over. You know what, though, it doesn't stop me from fasting again when I really desire to come out ahead on something. Fasting has become a way of life for me. I usually go on a week or more fast several times a year.

Susie, 22-Year-Old- Woman on Her Fourth Fast
The last time I fasted, I really wanted to meet my soul mate, but that didn't happen. I'm not sure that was the right reason to go on a fast, but oh well. I did discover things about myself. However, that was probably contributing to my inability to make lasting relationships. I think I fear commitment, and I attract people who feel the same. So, I'm working on that— that, and my confidence. Fasting has helped me out a lot, and I plan on making fasting a part of my life from now on.

Brendon, 48-Year-Old-Man Who Tried to Fast Once
I tried it once, thinking that it would be a breeze. It wasn't! I guess food is more important to me than I thought. I wanted to fast for four days, but I didn't even last through 24 hours. I don't know if I'll do it again. I've just got a lot of other things going on now, and fasting doesn't quite fit into my schedule.

Max, 27-Year-Old-Man Who Is a Body Builder
Fasting is great. It's hard for me sometimes because I need to be careful and not burn through muscle. I don't usually fast for long, just a little to clear my skin. Bodybuilding takes its toll on your skin, and I've suffered from acne most of my life. I find that fasting helps to cleanse my skin and gives me more energy. I can also concentrate more on lifting after a fast. Yeah, I'd recommend it to someone who was looking for a way to remove the toxins from your body. It definitely works, but you have to drink a lot of water too.

Nicolas, 40-Year-Old Pastor
I fast because that is what God instructs us to do, and I feel there are many benefits to fasting. Not only does it cleanse the body and purify the mind, but it helps me, personally, to draw closer to God and have a better understanding of my purpose in life. After I fast, everything seems a little sharper in my mind. Nature is more colorful and inviting, I communicate with my friends, family, and congregation better, and I just feel closer to God. It can be a sacrifice to God, but he sacrificed for me and fasting is the least I can do. So, yes, I fast often, and especially when I am seeking God's grace and wisdom.

Catherine, 55-Year-Old-Widow Woman After Her First Fast

After my husband passed away, I couldn't seem to work through the depression and loneliness. A very close friend told me about her success with fasting, and I was intrigued. At first, I was skeptical, but the more I thought about it, the more I wondered if it would help me to process all that had happened. She was great about giving me guidance and telling me what to expect. I fasted for four days, and she was right there with me all the way. I'm not sure I would have been able to stick with it that long without her, but her encouragement and support gave me hope and understanding. Although I'm not entirely out of the woods, and there are days where I still feel the old negative emotions come back to haunt me, it's much better. I believe my next fast will help me even more.

Now that you have learned more about fasting, we hope that you will be well-prepared for your next fast. Thank you for downloading this book! I hope we have been able to help you to have a new perspective and broader expectation of what fasting can do for you.

The next step is to begin preparing for your next fast. Arm yourself with the tools we have given you in this book, and follow our *Six Steps to Safe Fasting* to maximize all the positives a fast can provide. Fasting is more than a physical or emotional experience; it is a spiritual one as well, so be prepared to grow in all areas of your life and change your perspective on the things that are real and significant.

Because you know more about fasting, don't expect your fasts from here on out to be a walk in the park. The strength of your purpose and resolve with give you the determination and perseverance to complete your fast and come out the other side a more insightful and appreciative person. When the fast is a particularly tough one, you can expect your rewards to be that much better. With each new fast and purpose, you move closer to a greater awareness of yourself and a better understanding of others.

We're so thankful that you decided to fast the "safe" way by practicing our *Six Steps to Safe Fasting*. To review, they are as follows.

1. Setting a Plan and Purpose
2. Commit to the Fast
3. Preparing Yourself Mentally for the Fast
4. Preparing Yourself Physically for the Fast
5. Staying Focused During the Fast
6. Breaking the Fast

Following the safe steps to fasting that you have read about in

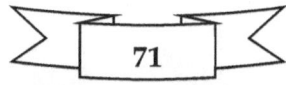

this book will assist you in maintaining an active, healthy body and mind both during and after your fast. Because you have learned to prepare adequately for your fast, you will have avoided some of the dangers and discomforts that many people suffer who are perhaps ill-suited or ignorant of the safe and efficient method of fasting.

After helping yourself maintain a healthier, stronger, more energetic body through fasting, you'll be eager to share your knowledge with others. Your friends and family members are going to see the change in you. They'll notice your positive attitude and renewed spirit to experience life to its fullest. You can choose to keep all you've learned a secret, or you can help them to experience what you have. One way to help them is to talk about what you learned when practicing our six steps.

Finally, if you enjoyed this book, then I'd like to ask you for a favor; would you be kind enough to leave a review for this book on Amazon? It'd be greatly appreciated!
Click here to leave a review for this book on Amazon!
Thank you and good luck on all your future fasts!

www.ingramcontent.com/pod-product-compliance
Lightning Source LLC
Chambersburg PA
CBHW020902310526
45786CB00018B/1529